How Do I Survive on Hemodialysis?

Philip J. Tuso, MD

authorHOUSE™

1663 LIBERTY DRIVE, SUITE 200
BLOOMINGTON, INDIANA 47403
(800) 839-8640
WWW.AUTHORHOUSE.COM

First published by AuthorHouse 4/5/2006

ISBN: 1-4208-3675-7 (sc)

Library of Congress Control Number: 2005902596

Printed in the United States of America
Bloomington, Indiana

This book is printed on acid-free paper.

Disclaimer

This book was written to help individuals with kidney failure understand how to survive on dialysis. The creator of this book does not warrant or assume any legal liability or responsibility for the accuracy, completeness, or usefulness of any information contained in this book.

The author of this book does not endorse or recommend any commercial products, processes, or services mentioned in this book. The views and opinions of the author expressed in this book do not necessarily state or reflect those of your health care professional team, kidney specialist, or your primary care physician.

It is not the intention of the author of this book to provide specific medical advice but rather to provide users with information to help individuals with kidney failure better understand their health issues and their diagnosis of kidney disease. Specific medical advice is not being provided. The author urges you to consult with a qualified physician for diagnosis and for answers to your personal questions.

This book is dedicated to the people of the Southern California Permanente Group Renal Management of the Antelope Valley.

Mary Mosser

Michal Sharabi

Katherine Dirden

Espie Abueg

Hong-Diep Nguyen

You have made me a better person.

You have made our patients better people.

You have made the world a better place to live.

Thank you for all your hard work.

SERVE Forward.

Table of Contents

Introduction

A. Kidney failure facts:

- One out of one thousand (1:1000) Americans have kidney failure.

- Medicare cost for treatment of kidney failure is approximately $20 billion per year.

- Medicare cost for each kidney failure patient is approximately $50,000 per year.

- One out of five (20%) Americans on dialysis will die each year.

B. Four jobs of the kidneys:

1. Kidneys eliminate waste products from our bodies.

   - Digestion and absorption of food produces nutrients and waste products.

   - Nutrients are used to keep our bodies healthy.

   - Waste products need to be eliminated on a daily basis to maintain good health.

   - In kidney failure, accumulation of waste products leads to loss of appetite, nausea and vomiting.

2. Kidneys remove extra minerals (potassium and phosphorus) from our body.

   - In kidney failure, excess potassium can cause sudden death.

    – In kidney failure, excess phosphorus can cause itchy skin and calcification of blood vessels.

3. Kidneys remove excess water and salt from our bodies.

    – In kidney failure, excess body salt and water may lead to elevated blood pressure and heart failure.

4. Kidneys produce two hormones called Vitamin D and Erythropoietin (EPO).

    – In kidney failure, lack of Vitamin D leads to bone pain and fractures.

    – In kidney failure, lack of EPO leads to anemia (low blood counts).

C. Hemodialysis:

1. Hemodialysis is the use of an artificial kidney to remove waste products, toxins, salt, and excess water from the blood.

2. People with kidney failure require hemodialysis to maintain life.

3. In general, the more compliant you are to your dialysis therapy the better you will feel and the longer you will live.

D. How to use this book?

1. Read each chapter slowly and if you do not understand a particular concept ask your physician or health care team member for advice.

2. Try to understand the key concept presented in each chapter and plan a course of action that will allow you to improve your measurable outcomes and increase you likelihood of living a longer and healthier life.

3. Each chapter is divided into the following sections to help you easily understand the material.

   - **Facts:** Interesting facts about the topic of discussion.

   - **Action items:** Easy steps you can take to increase your likelihood of survival on dialysis.

   - **Helpful chart:** Easy to read chart that gives you information to help you implement action items.

   - **Bottom line:** One or two sentence summary of the most important lesson to be learned from each chapter.

   Dialysis therapy is not the end of life.
   Dialysis therapy is the beginning of a new life.

I. Adjust all medications for kidney failure

- **Facts:**

  1. Many medications are metabolized by the body and excreted from the body by the kidneys.

  2. In kidney failure, medications that are usually excreted by the kidneys may accumulate in the body and cause serious side effects.

- **Action items:**

  1. Inform all health care providers that you have kidney disease.

  2. Keep a list of your medications with you at all times.

  3. In your list of medications include all of the following:
     - Name of medication.
     - Dosage of medication.
     - How medication is to be administered.
     - Frequency of medication administration.

       Example: labetalol 200 mg by mouth, twice per day

  4. Assure that all your medications have been adjusted for kidney failure.

- **Helpful chart:**

Medications that may require dose modification in kidney failure	
Medication	**Examples**
Heart drugs	digoxin
Antibiotics	penicillin, ciprofloxacin, sulfa, nitrofurantoin
Anti-viral	acyclovir
Anti-fungal	fluconazole
Anti-gout	allopurinol

Medications to avoid in kidney failure	
Medication	**Examples**
Anti-ulcer	cimetidine
Stool softeners	all products containing phosphate, magnesium, or aluminum
Diuretics (water pills)	potassium sparing diuretics
Pain Medications	nonsteroidal anti-inflammatory drugs
Radiology	dyes used for radiology and heart studies

- **Bottom line:**

  Inform all health care providers you have kidney disease.

II.   Avoid inadequate dialysis treatments

- **Facts:**
  1. **Adequate** dialysis means that the dialysis treatments you are receiving at the dialysis unit are **sufficient** to maintain life.

  2. **Inadequate** dialysis means that the dialysis treatments you are receiving at the dialysis unit are **insufficient** to maintain life.

  3. Dialysis adequacy is determined by calculating your Urea Reduction Ratio (URR). URR is determined by taking samples of blood before and after your dialysis treatment and sending samples for measurement of a kidney waste product called urea.

  4. Complications from inadequate dialysis:
     - Higher than normal death rate.
     - Increased number of days per year spent in the hospital.
     - Build up of kidney toxins that may lead to:
       - Shortness of breath.
       - Loss of appetite.
       - Feeling tired all the time.

- **Action items:**
  1. Three ways to increase dialysis adequacy:

- Increase time on dialysis.

- Increase blood flow rate through your artery vein access or catheter during dialysis.

- Increase size of membrane used for dialysis.

2. Do not miss any dialysis treatments.

3. Do not decrease the time you spend on dialysis.

- **Helpful chart:**

Urea Reduction Ratio or URR

- URR is a formula used to calculate adequacy of dialysis.
 	
 - URR equals the urea concentration in the blood at the beginning of dialysis (urea pre) minus the urea concentration in the blood at the end of dialysis (urea post) divided by the urea concentration in the blood at beginning of dialysis (urea pre).
 	
 - URR = urea pre - urea post/urea pre x 100 = % URR
 	
 - Example:
 	
   ❑ A dialysis patient is determined to have a urea concentration in the blood of 100 mg/dl before dialysis and a urea concentration in the blood of 30 mg/dl at the end of dialysis. What is this patient's URR?
 	
   ❑ URR = 100 - 30/100 = 70/100 x 100 = 70%

- **Bottom line:**

  Be compliant with your dialysis treatment regimen to assure adequate dialysis therapy and a Urea Reduction Ratio greater than 70%.

III. Avoid excessive weight gain

- **Facts:**

  1. When kidney function decreases, water consumed in our diet may not be removed by the kidneys and may remain in the body.

  2. Excess fluid in the body may cause:
     - Swelling of the ankles, skin, hands, and eyes
     - High blood pressure (excess fluid in blood vessels)
     - Congestive heart failure (excess fluid in heart and lungs)

  3. Drinking too much fluid between dialysis sessions can result in excessive weight gain. The amount of fluid gained can be determined by subtracting your weight before dialysis from your weight at the end of dialysis.

  4. Your weight at the end of dialysis is considered your dry weight because it represents the weight in which excess fluid has been completely removed from your body.

  5. Your weight gain could be considered excessive if you gain more than **three kg** of water weight between dialysis treatments.

  6. In kidney failure, hemodialysis may be the only effective way to remove excess fluid from the body.

- **Action items:**

    1. Understand the concept of dry weight and accurately measure your weight before and after each dialysis treatment.

    2. Do not gain more the 3 kg (or approximately 6 pounds) of fluid weight between dialysis treatments.

    3. Do not consume more than 6 cups or 48 ounces of total fluid per day between dialysis treatments.

    4. If you still make urine, your fluid intake per day should not exceed 6 cups of fluid plus your urine output. For example, if your urine output is 2 cups per day then your daily fluid intake should not exceed 8 cups per day (6 cups + 2 cups = 8 cups).

    5. Do not use dialysis fluid removal as a substitute for **not** monitoring the amount of fluid you consume between dialysis treatments.

        – **Sixty percent (60%)** of your total body weight is water. Most of your body water is inside your cells. Water outside your cells is located between cells and inside your blood vessels (arteries and veins). Only water inside your blood vessels is accessible to fluid being removed during dialysis.

        – The total amount of water in your blood vessels is about **six percent (6%)** of your total body weight.

        – Trying to remove water from your body greater than the amount of water in your blood vessels can be dangerous to your health and can cause cramping, nausea, vomiting, and low blood pressure.

- **Helpful chart:**

Fluid measurement tool		
Cup (s)	Ounces (oz)	Milliliters (ml)
1 cup	= 8oz	= 240 ml
2 cups	= 16oz	= 480 ml
3 cups	= 24oz	= 720 ml
4 cups	= 32oz	= 920 ml
5 cups	= 40oz	= 1200 ml
6 cups	**= 48oz**	**= 1400 ml**

Average fluid weight gain should not exceed blood vessel (artery and veins) water weight (kg)	
The amount of water in your blood vessels is approximately six percent of your total body weight.	
Weight (kg)	**Blood vessel water (estimate)**
100 kg	6 liters or 6 kg
90 kg	5.4 liters or 5.4 kg
80 kg	4.8 liters or 4.8 kg
70 kg	4.2 liters or 4.2 kg
60 kg	3.6 liters or 3.6 kg
50 kg	3.0 liters or 3.0 kg

- **Bottom line:**

  Unless otherwise instructed by your physician, do not gain more than 3 kg of fluid weight between hemodialysis treatments.

IV.   Avoid excessive sodium intake

- **Facts:**

  1. Sodium is a mineral or electrolyte that is involved in both electrical and cellular functions in the body.

  2. Normal kidneys remove excess sodium from the body and excrete the excess sodium into the urine.

  3. When kidney function decreases, sodium consumed in our diet is not removed by the kidneys and may remain in the body.

  4. Excess sodium in the body is associated with water retention and secondary swelling of extremities often called edema.

  5. Excess sodium in the body can cause increased thirst, tissue swelling, high blood pressure, and heart failure.

  6. Most people with kidney failure should be on a low sodium diet. A low sodium diet means you can consume about 2 grams (2000 mg) of sodium per day.

- **Action items:**

  1. Maintain a low sodium diet

     - 2 grams or 2000 mg of sodium per day

  2. Understand the amount of sodium in food.

  3. Avoid extra sodium in your diet if you are short of breath or observe swelling of your legs or hands.

4. Remember that water goes where sodium goes.

5. Always seek medical attention if you are short of breath.

- **Helpful chart:**

Sodium content of common foods	
Food	**Sodium (mg)**
One teaspoon table salt	2000 mg (2 grams)
One slice of lunch meat	300 mg
One hot dog	500 mg
One cup of soup	900 mg
One pickle (large)	1430 mg
One large slice of pizza	600 mg
One diet soda (12 ounces)	75 mg

- **Bottom line:**

Unless otherwise instructed by your physician, avoid consuming more than 2,000 mg or 2 grams of sodium per day while on long term dialysis therapy.

V.   Avoid low albumin levels

- **Facts:**

    1. Serum albumin is a protein in blood that is made in the liver and important for normal body function.

    2. Protein is used for growth and building of muscles, maintenance and repair of all body tissues, and maintenance and repair of your immune system.

    3. Low serum albumin is called malnutrition and can result in poor healing and decreased immunity.

    4. An abnormal immune system may result in an increased risk for infections, inflammation, and heart disease.

    5. Low serum albumin levels are associated with a high death rate.

    6. Increasing the amount of protein we consume in our diet can help to raise albumin levels in our blood.

    7. The recommended amount of protein people with kidney failure should consume per day to keep their bodies healthy is approximately 1.5 grams of protein per kg body weight.

    8. Meat and eggs are good sources of protein but can only be consumed in moderation because these nutritional supplements contain large amounts of cholesterol.

9. Protein supplements (designed specifically for people with kidney failure) and non-yolk eggs are excellent low cholesterol sources of protein.

- **Action items:**

   1. Consider supplementing your diet with protein nutritional supplements if your blood albumin levels are consistently lower than normal. Examples include:

      - Protein powder

      - Protein drinks

      - Protein bars

   2. Most over-the-counter nutritional supplements are not safe for people with kidney failure. Check with your physician or dialysis unit dietitian for a list of protein supplements that are safe for people with kidney failure.

   3. If your blood albumin levels are consistently lower than normal (less than 4.0 g/dl), ask your physician about taking medications that may raise your low albumin levels by reducing inflammation in your body.

      - Daily aspirin (anti-inflammatory)

      - Cholesterol lowering drugs (statins)

      - Vitamins (folic acid and Vitamin B-12)

      - Fish oil tablets (omega 3 fatty acids).

4. If your blood albumin levels are consistently lower than normal, ask your physician about taking medications that may treat conditions that prevent absorption of proteins from your diet:

   – Nausea and vomiting

   – Heart burn or indigestion

   – Depression (loss of appetite)

- **Helpful chart:.**

Daily protein requirement by weight		
Weight		Protein requirement
Kg	Pounds	Grams per day
50	110	75
60	132	90
70	154	105
80	176	120
90	198	135
100	220	150
110	242	165
120	264	180
130	286	195

Grams of protein per unit dose for common sources of protein and commonly used nutritional supplements		
Source	**Protein per unit dose**	
Meat	7	grams of protein per ounce
Eggs	7	grams of protein per egg
No yolk eggs	25	grams of protein per cup
Protein powder	5	grams of protein per scoop
Protein drink	15	grams of protein per can
Protein bars	15	grams of protein per bar

- **Bottom line:**

  Unless otherwise instructed by your physician, try to consume at least 1.5 grams per kilogram (kg) of protein per day to maintain a serum albumin level greater than 4.0 g/dl.

VI.   Avoid anemia

- **Facts:**
  1. Anemia is defined as having less than a normal number of red blood cells or less than normal hemoglobin in the blood.

  2. Hemoglobin is a red pigment that gives the red color to red blood cells and to blood. Hemoglobin is the key chemical compound that combines with oxygen from the lungs and carries the oxygen from the lungs to cells throughout the body. Oxygen is essential for cells to produce energy.

  3. When hemoglobin is low, oxygen transport through the body is low.

  4. The person with anemia is under-oxygenated and may complain about feeling tired, and becoming short of breath with exercise.

  5. Anemia is caused by low levels of iron in the blood and/or a decrease in production of a hormone called EPO.

     - People who are iron deficient usually have blood tests that show their total body iron stores have been depleted.

     - Two tests commonly used to determine body iron stores are transferrin saturation and blood ferritin levels.

- A person is considered iron deficient if their transferrin saturation level is less than 20% and a blood ferritin level is less than 100 ng/ml.

- **Action items:**

  1. Record and review with your physician your hemoglobin levels monthly.

  2. Understand that you may be given EPO or iron during dialysis to help your body produce red blood cells.

  3. Understand that your hemoglobin goal is 11 gm/dl.

  4. Understand that high blood pressure, headache and/or flu-like symptoms may be side effects of EPO.

- **Helpful chart:**

Anemia Terms
Red Blood Cells (RBC): - Cells that carry oxygen in your blood.
Hemoglobin (Hgb): - Protein in red blood cells that binds oxygen.
Hematocrit (Hct): - Percent of red blood cells in the blood.

- **Bottom line:**

  Unless otherwise instructed by your physician, try to maintain a blood hemoglobin level greater than 11 g/dl.

VII. Avoid bone disease

- **Facts:**

  1. The normal kidney makes active Vitamin D that is required to keep your body healthy. When the kidney is diseased, active Vitamin D is no longer produced.

  2. A deficiency of Vitamin D results in a cascade of events that lowers serum calcium levels.

  3. As serum calcium levels fall, the body secretes a hormone called parathyroid hormone (PTH), whose main purpose is to normalize blood calcium levels.

  4. PTH is the most important endocrine regulator of calcium and phosphorus concentration in body fluid. PTH is secreted from cells of the parathyroid glands in the neck and finds its major target cells in the bones and kidneys. PTH binds to cells in the kidneys and causes them to produce Vitamin D.

  5. When calcium levels return to normal, excess Vitamin D goes to the parathyroid gland and signals to the parathyroid gland to stop making PTH.

  6. When Vitamin D levels are low in kidney failure, PTH levels remain elevated and cause a gradual breakdown of bone and a constant release of calcium and phosphorus into the blood.

  7. A patient with kidney disease is unable to excrete excess phosphorus in the urine so phosphorus levels in the blood can rise to dangerous levels.

8. Excess phosphorus in the blood binds with calcium in the blood and forms bone like tissue (calcification) in joints and blood vessels.

9. Calcification of your blood vessels may result in vascular diseases like stroke or heart attack.

- **Action items:**

  1. Lower blood levels of phosphorus by avoiding foods high in phosphorus.

  2. Take medications that bind phosphorus in your food to prevent phosphorus absorption in the gastrointestinal tract. Examples are shown below. Ask your physician which type of medication is best for you.

     Examples of commonly used phosphate binders
     - calcium carbonate
     - calcium acetate
     - sevelamar

  3. Understand that your physician may try to give you intravenous Vitamin D during dialysis to suppress secretion of PTH.

- **Helpful chart:**

Foods that are high in phosphorus (foods to avoid)
Dairy products: - milk, cheese, yogurt, cream soup
Fruits and vegetables: - asparagus, peas, mushrooms, corn, beans
Breads: - muffins, pancakes, waffles, whole wheat bread, pizza
Nuts and seeds
Chocolate and cocoa
Colas and beer

- **Bottom line:**

  Unless otherwise instructed by your physician, try to maintain a serum phosphorus level less than 5.5 mg/dl and a parathyroid hormone level less than 180 pg/ml.

VIII. Avoid high potassium levels

- **Facts:**

    1. Potassium is a mineral or electrolyte that is involved in both electrical and cellular functions in the body. Potassium is found in human cells and most foods. Potassium plays a role in keeping your heartbeat regular and your muscles working properly.

    2. It is the job of the kidneys to keep the right amount of potassium in your body. When kidneys fail, the body has difficulty eliminating potassium.

    3. High levels of potassium in your blood can cause your heart to stop beating and result in sudden death.

    4. Potassium can be removed from your body during hemodialysis.

- **Action items:**

    1. Understand that the recommended daily allowance for potassium for people with kidney disease is 2 grams (2,000 mg) per day.

    2. Never miss or cut short your dialysis treatments.

    3. Avoid medications that cause high potassium levels.

    4. Avoid foods that are very high in potassium and can acutely raise your blood potassium levels and

result in serious complications. Examples include tomatoes, bananas, oranges and potatoes.

- **Helpful chart:**

Foods that are high in potassium (foods to avoid)
Salt substitutes: - potassium chloride
Dairy products: - milk, yogurt, cheeses
Whole grains: - breads, cereals, muffins
Starchy vegetables: - **potatoes**, dried beans, yams, winter squash
Other vegetables: - **tomatoes**, broccoli, peas, lima beans, spinach
Fruits: - **bananas**, **oranges**, citrus fruits, apricots

- **Bottom line:**

High blood potassium levels can cause sudden death. Avoid blood potassium levels greater then 5.5 meq/L.

IX. Control risk factors for heart attack

- **Facts:**
  1. LDL or low density lipoprotein is that portion of total cholesterol that is considered bad cholesterol.

     – LDL is the bad cholesterol because it takes cholesterol from the liver and deposits cholesterol on the blood vessels in the heart.

     – High levels of LDL cholesterol are associated with a high death rate secondary to heart attack.

  2. HgbA1C is a blood test that is used to monitor long term blood sugar control in people with diabetes mellitus.

     – Elevated HgbA1C levels means your diabetes is poorly controlled.

     – Low HgbA1C levels means you do not have diabetes mellitus or that your diabetes mellitus is under good control.

  3. High blood pressure is an independent risk factor for kidney disease, heart disease, and stroke.

     – Two or more medications are usually required to control high blood pressure in kidney disease.

- **Action items:**
  1. Control LDL cholesterol levels

     – Follow a low cholesterol diet.

- Take cholesterol-lowering medications if your LDL cholesterol levels are elevated.

- Ask your physician to monitor your LDL cholesterol levels.

2. Control diabetes mellitus

- Follow an 1800-calorie American Diabetic Diet.

- Take insulin and/or medications as needed to maintain blood sugar levels in normal range.

- Monitor blood glucose levels frequently and inform your physician if blood sugar levels are persistently elevated.

3. Control blood pressure

- Follow a 2-gram low sodium diet.

- Monitor blood pressure closely during dialysis therapy.

- Take blood pressure medications if you have high blood pressure.

- Ask you physician to consider adjusting your blood pressure medications if your blood pressure is not normal.

- **Helpful chart:**

Goals to decrease risk of heart attack
LDL or bad cholesterol level less than 100 mg/dl
HgBA1C level less than 7%
Blood pressure less than 130/80 mmHg

- **Bottom line:**

  Uncontrolled diabetes mellitus, high blood pressure and high cholesterol are associated with early death in people with kidney failure.

X.   Avoid dialysis catheters

- **Facts:**

    1. Your vascular access is your "lifeline" for survival.

        – Your vascular access is the part of your body where blood is removed during dialysis. Examples include artery vein fistula, artery vein graft and a dialysis catheter. Dialysis catheters can be temporary (usually do not require a visit to the operating room for insertion) or permanent (usually require a visit to the operating room for insertion).

        – Caring for your vascular access is vital for your long term health and survival.

        – Individuals with fistulas and grafts have a lower death rate than individuals with catheters.

    2. Complications associated with dialysis catheters include infection, clotting, and poor blood flows.

        – Risk factors for dialysis catheter infections include diabetes mellitus, low albumin, and nasal carriage of bacteria that are known to cause catheter infections.

        – Severe catheter infections may cause infections of the heart, infections of the bone, infections of the spinal cord, and death.

- **Action items:**

  1. Try to avoid dialysis catheters.

  2. Request an artery vein fistula as your first choice for dialysis access.

  3. Protect the extremity where your artery vein access is located (left or right upper extremity).

     - No needle sticks (blood draws) of your access extremity except by your dialysis team.

     - No blood pressure measurements of your access extremity.

  4. Prevent artery vein access or catheter related infections

     - Keep your access clean and only use your access for dialysis.

     - Inform dentists and physicians you have kidney failure and need antibiotic prophylaxis to prevent access related infections associated with dental and surgical procedures.

     - Alert any health care provider if you have fever, chills, or access skin redness (signs of access related infection).

     - Assure all antibiotics used to treat infections are adjusted for kidney failure.

- **Helpful chart:**

Different types of hemodialysis access

- Dialysis catheter: sterile tubing inserted into a vein in the neck, chest wall or groin to allow blood access for hemodialysis

- Artery vein graft: surgical connection of an artery to a vein using artificial tubing (graft) usually in the arm to allow blood access for hemodialysis

- Artery vein fistula: surgical connection directly between an artery and vein to allow access for hemodialysis

---

Risk of infection with different types of hemodialysis access

Type of Access	Infection Risk
- Temporary catheter	Extremely high
- Permanent catheter	Very high
- Artery vein graft	Low
- Artery vein fistula	Very low

Antibiotic prophylaxis for dental or surgical procedures

1. All hemodialysis patients require antibiotic prophylaxis before dental and surgical procedures to prevent access related infections of catheters, artery vein grafts, and artery vein fistulas.

2. Standard general antibiotic prophylaxis can be given orally or intravenously (IV) to prevent access related infections:

   − Standard oral general antibiotic prophylaxis

      □ No penicillin allergy: amoxicillin 2000 mg orally one hour before procedure.

      □ Penicillin allergy options:

         ▪ clindamycin 600 mg orally one hour before procedure -OR-

         ▪ cephalexin 2000 mg (2.0 g) orally one hour before procedure -OR-

         ▪ azithromycin 500 mg orally one hour before the procedure

   − Standard intravenous general antibiotic prophylaxis

      □ No penicillin allergy: cefazolin 1.0 g IV one hour before procedure

      □ Penicillin allergy: vancomycin 1.0 g IV one hour before the procedure.

- **Bottom line:**

  Artery vein fistulas for dialysis are associated with a very low infection rate and a very low death rate.

XI. Avoid preventable infections

- **Facts:**

  1. Community acquired infections can be prevented by immunization.

  2. Each year, thousands of kidney disease patients die from pneumonia and influenza.

  3. Hepatitis means inflammation of the liver. Hepatitis B virus infections are usually caused by exposure to blood of someone with Hepatitis B viral infection (needle stick or blood transfusion).

     – Because kidney disease patients are at risk to receive a blood transfusion, all patients with kidney disease are immunized with a vaccine that will decrease their chance of developing Hepatitis B infection.

     – After receiving appropriate Hepatitis B vaccination, blood tests are performed to determine if appropriate antibodies have formed to protect the patient from hepatitis B viral infection.

     – After antibodies are formed to hepatitis B virus, you will have developed immunity that may prevent you from developing liver disease from hepatitis B virus exposure.

- **Action items:**

  1. Prevent pneumonia.

2. Prevent the flu.

3. Prevent hepatitis.

- **Helpful chart:**

Vaccinations schedules	
Pneumonia	Every five years
Flu	Every Fall
Hepatitis B	0, 1, 2 and 6 months

- **Bottom line:**

Vaccinations save lives.

XII: Monitor measurable outcomes

- **Facts:**

  1. Effectiveness in achieving your goal for surviving on dialysis can be established by defining specific goals and monitoring your progress using monthly measurable outcomes.

  2. Data relating to your outcomes can be used to ascertain to what extent each goal has been achieved.

  3. Data on the effectiveness of your treatment for kidney failure are performed on dialysis patients monthly.

  4. Laboratory tests and other data measurements are obtained monthly and reviewed by your health care team. Adjustments will be made in your treatment regimen based on your monthly test results.

- **Action items:**

  1. Review your laboratory test results with your dialysis team on a monthly basis.

  2. Understand how you can improve all your measurable outcomes.

  3. Understand the reasoning for all medication and treatment adjustments based on your monthly measurable outcomes.

• Helpful chart

Measurable Outcomes	Goals
I. Medication Management	All medications adjusted for kidney failure
II. Dialysis Adequacy	URR > 70%
III. Weight Gain Management	Pre dialysis weight minus dry weight is < 3 kg
IV. Salt Intake Management	Salt intake < 2,000 mg/day
V. Albumin Management	Albumin level > 4 g/dl
VI. Anemia Management	Hemoglobin > 11 g/dl
VII. Bone Management	Phosphorus < 5.5 mg/dl PTH < 180 pg/ml
VIII. Potassium Management	Potassium < 5.5 meq/L
IX. Heart Attack Risk Factors	LDL <100 mg/dl HgbA1C < 7% BP < 130/80 mmHg
X. Dialysis Catheters	Artery Vein Fistula as preferred access for hemodialysis
XI. Vaccinations	Pneumonia, Flu and Hepatitis B
URR = Urea Reduction Ratio	
PTH = parathyroid hormone	
BP = blood pressure	

Management of Measurable Outcomes Not Meeting Goal	
Measurable Outcomes	**Management**
I. No medication list	Make a medication list and review with your physician.
II. URR < 70%	Increase time on dialysis per physician.
III. Excess weight gain	Monitor fluid intake.
IV. Excess sodium intake	Monitor sodium intake.
V. Albumin level < 4 g/dl	Protein supplementation.
VI. Hemoglobin < 11 g/dl	EPO dose adjustment and intravenous iron per physician.
VII. PTH > 180 pg/ml	Low phosphorus diet. Vitamin D dose adjustment per physician.
VIII. Potassium > 5.5 meq/L	Low potassium diet.
IX Heart Disease Risk Factors	
– LDL > 100 mg/dl	Adjust cholesterol medications per physician.
– HgbA1C > 7%	Adjust diabetes mellitus medications per physician.
– BP > 130/80 mmHg	Adjust blood pressure medication per physician.
X. Dialysis Catheter	Vascular surgery referral per physician.
XI. No vaccinations	Vaccinations per physician.

- **Bottom line**

   Your survival on dialysis depends on your ability to have measurable outcomes that are within normal range for people with chronic renal failure.

Conclusion:

- **Facts:**

  1. Survival on dialysis can be improved by compliance to treatment regimens, diet, and medications.

  2. Reduction in risk factors for coronary artery disease can significantly decrease the likelihood of dying from a heart attack.

- **Action items:**

  1. Be in control

     - Take control of your diet and your disease.

  2. Be courageous

     - Do not be afraid to learn new information.

  3. Be wise

     - Focus on monthly measurable outcomes.

  4. Be just

     - Work with your physician to adjust your treatment plan based on your measurable outcomes.

- **Bottom line:**

  Chronic dialysis is a journey not a destination.

Resources

1. Kidney Disease Quality Outcomes Initiative (NKF-K/DOQI)

   - Clinical Practice Guidelines for Hemodialysis Adequacy: update 2000. Am J Kidney Dis - 01-JAN-2001; 37(1 Suppl 1): S7-S64

   - Clinical Practice Guidelines for Vascular Access: update 2000. Am J Kidney Dis - 01-JAN-2001; 37(1 Suppl 1): S137-81

   - The National Kidney Foundation K/DOQI clinical practice guidelines for dietary protein intake for chronic dialysis patients. Kopple JD National Kidney Foundation K/DOQI Work Group - Am J Kidney Dis - 01-OCT-2001; 38(4 Suppl 1): S68-73

2. United States Renal Data System (USRDS). USRDS 2001 Annual Data Report: Atlas of End-Stage Renal Diseases in the United States. Bethesda, Md: National Institutes of Health, National Institute of Diabetes and Digestive and Kidney Diseases; 2001.

3. Brenner & Rector's The Kidney, 7th ed. Copyright © 2004 Elsevier

Resources

American Association of Kidney Patients
3505 East Frontage Road
Suite 315
Tampa, FL 33607
Phone: 1-800-749-2257 or (813) 636-8100
Email: info@aakp.org
Internet: www.aakp.org

Life Options Rehabilitation Program
c/o Education Institute Inc.
414 D'Onofrio Drive
Suite 200
Madison, WI 53711-1074
Phone: 1-800-468-7777 or (608) 232-2333
Email: lifeoptions@medmed.com
Internet: www.lifeoptions.org
www.kidneyschool.org

National Kidney Foundation Inc.
30 East 33rd Street
New York, NY 10016
Phone: 1-800-622-9010 or (212) 889-2210
Email: info@kidney.org
Internet: www.kidney.org

Foundation to Improve Renal Nutrition (FIRN)

Kidney disease affects one out of every ten Americans. Kidney failure, which requires dialysis therapy or renal transplantation to maintain life, affects one out of every thousand Americans. One out of two patients who are malnourished and on dialysis will die each year.

The Foundation to Improve Renal Nutrition is a non-profit public benefit corporation started in January of 2004. Your donation to FIRN will help educate individuals with kidney disease, and their families, on the importance of nutrition in preventing and treating the many complications associated with kidney disease. More importantly, your donation will provide protein nutritional supplements for malnourished patients with kidney disease who cannot afford them.

With your help, we can eliminate malnutrition in kidney disease and help individuals with kidney failure live longer and healthier lives.

For more information, please visit the FIRN web site @ http://firnav.org

SERVE Forward

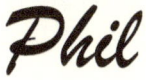

Books by Philip J. Tuso, MD, FACP

Who Stole My Kidneys?

*A book about saving kidneys
and saving lives in America.*

It is estimated that 20 million Americans have chronic kidney disease. Americans with kidney disease have a very high mortality rate over a five-year period—ranging from about 20% for Americans with mild or moderate kidney disease to almost 50% in Americans with severe kidney disease.

In this book, four imaginary characters are used to exemplify how virtues or character strengths determine the outcome of those who developed kidney disease. Using these characters, the book illustrates how having an illness like chronic kidney disease may involve facing new situations, complicated problems, challenges, and obstacles that sometimes could (or can) have no right or easy answers.

In this book, you will see that being proactive can prevent kidney damage and early death. The educational material in this book is a survival manual and a must read for all individuals with kidney disease.

SERVE Forward

A story about how serving others can help you
live a more meaningful and successful life.

Greatness in life consists not of doing great deeds with great means but of doing great deeds with little means. Serving does not require great resources. All it requires is the willingness and desire to serve. We can all be great because we can all learn how to serve.

In this book, you will see that to serve means to be wise, fair, strong, and sincere. Clarifying the concept of service helps people understand the long-term benefits of a service-driven life. This concept is a grounded philosophy that can apply to all walks of life. This book will be helpful to individuals who are interested in using the serve forward philosophy to help them live a healthier life and build meaningful relationships at work and at home.

About the author

Philip Tuso, MD, is a board certified nephrologist who has received numerous awards and held many administrative positions before being appointed Physician Director of the Fresenius Medical Care Dialysis Unit in Lancaster, California. Over the past year, Dr. Tuso has focused on efforts to develop a population care management program to help improve measurable outcomes for individuals with chronic kidney disease. He is the founder and president of a non-profit organization called the Foundation to Improve Renal Nutrition, whose mission is to increase public awareness of kidney disease and raise funds to supply nutritional supplements to malnourished individuals with kidney failure.

www.ingramcontent.com/pod-product-compliance
Lightning Source LLC
Chambersburg PA
CBHW021926170526
45157CB00005B/2202